Effectiveness and Safety of Cholesterol Lowering Dietary Supplements

by

Lance Fontenot, Ph.D.

About the Author

Lance Fontenot, Ph.D. is an environmental toxicologist with more than 20 years of experience focused on toxicity assessment and human health and ecological risk assessment. Research and applied environmental consulting experience have included conducting toxicity assessments of various chemicals, developing toxicity criteria protective of human and ecological health, and studies on the use of various organisms as bioindicators of environmental contamination. My belief is that health can be optimized through proper nutrition and dietary supplements. However, there is a lack of translation of the scientific literature on dietary supplements to actionable health choices. The topic of high cholesterol is personal to me and was the impetus for the development of this book.

Medical Disclaimer

Views or opinions presented in this book are solely those of the author and do not represent those of any medical organization, state or federal agency involved with dietary supplements. The information provided in this book is intended to provide recent (as of 2018), accurate science-based information as reference material only and not as medical or professional advice. The objective of this book is to provide consumers with the information to make informed decisions regarding dietary supplements and claims of effectiveness and safety. The information provided in this book should not be used as a substitute for any treatment that has been prescribed by your personal doctor.
The information presented here is offered for educational purposes only and should not be construed as personal *medical advice*. This information is not a substitute for health care provided by your personal medical or other health care providers. For those people who are currently taking medication for the treatment of high cholesterol, that treatment should continue unless otherwise directed by your personal physician.

While the author has attempted to utilize best efforts in preparing this book, the author makes no expressed representation or warranty with respect to the accuracy, applicability, or completeness of the contents of this book. The author disclaims all responsibility for any liability, loss or risk, personal or other, incurred as a result, directly or indirectly, of the use and application of the contents of this book. Whenever there is any doubt about your personal medical condition, a health care professional should be consulted, and the contents of this book should not be relied upon.

Any products mentioned are used as example solely for illustration. The mention by name or picture is *not to endorse or discredit* a product.

Conflict of Interest

I have no conflicts of interest that are relevant to the contents of this book. I have not received any compensation from any sources to write this book. The evaluations and information presented herein are my own opinion, are impartial, and based on the available scientific evidence regarding the effectiveness and safety of cholesterol lowering dietary supplements. I think it is also important to disclose that I have high cholesterol and have used various dietary supplements to control my own cholesterol levels. I have also suffered from SAMS but have been able to transition from statin drug therapy to dietary supplements and lifestyle changes. To date, I have been successful, but my cholesterol levels are never ideal.

Abbreviations and Acronyms

AHA = American Heart Association

CVD = cardiovascular disease

DHA = docosahexaenoic acid (omega-3 fatty acids)

EFSA = European Food Safety Authority

EPA = eicosapentaenoic acid (omega-3 fatty acids)

FDA = U.S. Food and Drug Administration

g = grams

HDL-C = high-density lipoprotein cholesterol ("good cholesterol")

LDL-C = low-density lipoprotein cholesterol ("bad cholesterol")

µg = micrograms

mg = milligram

mg/dl = milligrams per deciliter

SAMS = statin-associated muscle symptoms

TC = total cholesterol

TG = triglycerides

Table of Contents

Chapter 1: Introduction 1

Chapter 2: Lipid-lowering Mechanisms of Action 3

Chapter 3: Red Yeast Rice 6

Chapter 4: Bergamot 11

Chapter 5: Berberine 13

Chapter 6: Fish Oil 15

Chapter 7: Krill Oil 18

Chapter 8: Phytosterols 21

Chapter 9: Soluble Fiber 23

Chapter 10: Artichoke 26

Chapter 11: Garlic 28

Chapter 12: Rice Bran Oil 30

Chapter 13: Soy Protein 32

Chapter 14: Green Tea 35

Chapter 15: Chitosan 37

Chapter 16: Spirulina 39

Chapter 17: Probiotics 41

Chapter 18: Flaxseed 43

Chapter 19: Other Dietary Supplements with
Limited Effectiveness 45

Chapter 20: Summary and Recommended Approach 47

CHAPTER 1

Introduction

According to the American Heart Association (AHA), heart disease is the Number 1 global cause of death accounting for 17 million deaths per year. Almost 1 in 3 American adults have high cholesterol which is widely recognized as a risk factor for heart disease and is a modifiable cardiovascular risk factor. Dyslipidemia is the medical term for the elevation of lipids (e.g., triglycerides, cholesterol, and fat phospholipids in the blood) and is a major factor in cardiovascular disease. The standard medical treatment for dyslipidemia is lipid-lowering therapy. Typical drugs prescribed for treatment are referred to as statins and have side effects that are an issue for many people. LDL-C is the primary target for cholesterol lowering therapy as it is believed to be the major cause of atherosclerosis which is plaque buildup inside your arteries.

Naturally derived dietary supplements have been utilized as an alternative therapy to lower blood levels of total cholesterol (TC), improve the balance between low-density lipoprotein cholesterol (LDL-C; "bad cholesterol) and high-density lipoprotein (HDL-C; "good cholesterol"), and lower triglycerides (TG). However, there is no "magical" supplement that can replace regular exercise, healthy lifestyle choices, and a healthy, balanced diet to improve cholesterol levels.

Desirable Cholesterol Levels

Total Cholesterol	LDL-C	HDL-C	Triglycerides
<200 mg/dl	<100 mg/dl	>60 mg/dl	<150 mg/dl

From: Centers for Disease Control and Prevention

The objective of this book is to provide a review of the most promising dietary supplements that can be used for cholesterol control. This includes recent articles summarizing the results of clinical studies and expert opinions of the International Lipid Expert Panel, a multi-disciplinary group of worldwide experts focused on education and management of atherosclerosis, lipid disorders, and their resulting complications. There are other popular dietary supplements for cholesterol control that are not included due to lack of effectiveness or safety considerations. Each chapter of this book covers an individual dietary supplement and concisely summarizes the following information from the available scientific data:

> What is it?

> Effectiveness and Recommended Dose

> How does it work?

> Safety Concerns and Upper Limits

> Interactions with medications

> References

The individual dietary supplement chapters are presented in order of effectiveness. Safety information includes upper limits when available.

CHAPTER 2

Lipid-lowering Mechanisms of Action

Understanding the mechanism of action of a dietary supplement increases the possibility that it may be effective in lowering lipid levels. Dietary supplements without a defined mechanism of action do not have a scientific basis for proposed health benefits and effectiveness. For example, multivitamins have previously been thought to play a role in cardiovascular disease, but a clear mechanism of action was not defined. A recent study has demonstrated that taking multivitamins did not prevent heart attacks, strokes, or death from heart disease. This finding is consistent with guidelines from the AHA which do not recommend taking multivitamins to prevent cardiovascular disease.

Dietary supplements that are effective for lowering cholesterol have a mechanism of action that is specifically linked to a physiological process that reduces lipids. As elevated lipids are a known risk factor for heart disease, there is a clear linkage of the lipid-lowering mechanism to a health benefit.

The major categories of lipid-lowering mechanisms of action and the dietary supplements within these categories are:

1. Inhibition of Intestinal Cholesterol Absorption

    a. Phytosterols

    b. Soluble Fiber

    c. Chitosan

    d. Probiotics

2.   Inhibition of Liver Cholesterol Synthesis

   a.   Red Yeast Rice

   b.   Bergamot

   c.   Garlic

   d.   Flaxseed

3.   Enhancement of the Excretion of LDL-C

   a.   Berberine

   b.   Soy Protein

   c.   Green Tea

   d.   Mixed Mechanisms of Action

4.   Fish Oil

   a.   Krill Oil

   b.   Artichoke

   c.   Rice Bran Oil

   d.   Spirulina

While the focus of this book is on those supplements with demonstrated lipid-lowering effects, several dietary supplements also have additional positive effects on cardiovascular function. These include improvement of endothelial dysfunction and arterial stiffness in addition to anti-inflammatory and anti-oxidative properties. The development of cardiovascular disease is complex and there are still poorly understood areas including factors that affect disease progression and means of prevention and treatment.

References

Cicero, A. F., A. Colletti, G. Bajraktari, O. Descamps, D. M. Djuric, M. Ezhov, Z. Fras, N. Katsiki, M. Langlois, G. Latkovskis, et al. 2017. Lipid lowering nutraceuticals in clinical practice: position paper from an International Lipid Expert Panel. Archives of Medical Science 13:965–1005.

Jenkins, D.J., J. D. Spence, E. L. Giovannucci, et al. 2018. Supplemental Vitamins and Minerals for CVD Prevention and Treatment. *J Am Coll Cardiol* 2018; 71:2570-84.

Thaipitakwong, T. and P. Aramwit. 2017. A review of the efficacy, safety, and clinical implications of naturally derived dietary supplements for dyslipidemia. American Journal of Cardiovascular Drugs. 2017 Feb;17(1):27-35.

CHAPTER 3

Red Yeast Rice

What is it?

Red yeast rice (RYR) is obtained by the fermentation of yeast in rice. The primary active ingredients are called monacolins which have lipid lowering effects. Monacolin content can be as high as 1.9%. There are several types of monacolins present in RYR. Monacolin K has a nearly identical chemical structure to lovastatin, a prescription statin drug. There has been considerable controversy as to whether RYR should be regulated as a drug. The U.S. Food and Drug Administration (FDA) has removed some RYR supplements from the market because they contained lovastatin. Other ingredients of RYR include sterols, isoflavones, and unsaturated fatty acids which may also influence blood lipid levels.

Effectiveness and Recommended Dose

RYR has been shown to be effective in reducing levels of TC, LDL-C, and TG. HDL-C levels have not been shown to increase. RYR has also been effective and well tolerated in statin-intolerant patients.

Identifying a daily effective dose for RYR is difficult as there is considerable variation in the monacolin content among the available formulations of RYR. However, the study by Gordon et al. (2010) provides the monacolin content of several brands of RYR which can be used as an estimate. Note that even different lots of the same brand of RYR could vary significantly in monacolin content. Daily doses of monacolin K in randomized clinical trials ranged from 3 – 10 mg and reduced LDL-C levels by 15 to 25%. Daily doses of "total" RYR tested ranging from 1200 mg to 3600 mg in randomized clinical trials have been shown to be effective in lowering TC, TG (13 – 44%), and LDL-C (21 -32%). Some studies have shown that the effectiveness of RYR is comparable to statin drugs, especially in combination with fish oil and therapeutic lifestyle changes (e.g. diet and exercise). Note that RYR should be taken in divided doses to increase absorption and maintain a more constant level of monacolins. Additionally, due to the variability of the active components of RYR, regular blood testing of cholesterol levels should be done to ensure that the product is working and not causing any adverse effects.

How does it work?

RYR works by inhibiting the key enzyme involved in the natural synthesis of cholesterol. This results in a reduction of your body's natural production of cholesterol. This is a similar mechanism to statin prescription drugs. Oral bioavailability of lovastatin (Monacolin K) in RYR products appears to be high and may help explain the effectiveness of RYR considering the very low doses present.

Safety Concerns and Upper Limits

In general, serious side effects have not been reported in clinical trials. However, there can be significant safety concerns with RYR. As shown by the study conducted by Gordon et al. (2010), RYR can be contaminated with citrinin which is a mycotoxin formed during the fermentation process. I recommend avoiding the brands that were reported to contain citrinin. Some newer products indicate that their formulation is "citrinin free." The European Food Safety Authority (EFSA) has established an upper limit for citrinin of 20 ug/kg body weight per day. However, this level was based only on kidney toxicity and did not consider other potential toxic effects.

Monacolin Levels and Citrinin Content reported for Red Rice Yeast Products (Gordon et al. 2010)

Product	Total Monacolins (mg/cap)	Monacolin K (mg/cap)	Citrinin (µg/cap)
21st Century 100% Vegetarian RYR Extract	5.30	2.53	0.0
Atrium Chole-sterin RYR	2.16	1.02	0.0
Cholestene HPF RYR	4.18	1.74	0.0
Healthy America RYR	1.65	1.12	14.3
Natural Balance RYR Concentrated Extract	6.03	3.63	0.0
Naturals	0.31	0.10	114.2
Nature's Plus Herbal Actives RYR (1.7% total monacolins)	6.18	2.50	0.0
ResQ LDL-X	11.15	10.09	0.0
Schiff New RYR	1.60	0.99	57.5
Solaray RYR	3.97	2.66	0.0
VegLife 100% Vegan RYR	1.36	0.97	70.4
Walgreens Finest Natural RYR	6.13	3.12	0.0

Abbreviations: mg/cap = milligrams per capsule; µg/cap = micrograms per capsule

Interactions with medications

Because of the similarity in mechanism of action, RYR should not be taken at the same time as prescription statins. Other potential interactions (muscle effects) could occur if RYR is taken at the same time as grapefruit juice, cyclosporine, niacin, fibrates, coumarin, verapamil, antifungals, macrolides, nefazodone, and HIV protease inhibitors. Statin drugs also inhibit the production of Coenzyme Q-10 so it is recommended that this supplement should also be taken when using RYR. Some evidence also suggests that supplemental Coenzyme Q-10 might also help relieve any muscle weakness similar to that caused by statins. Additionally, RYR should only be taken when blood lipid levels, liver enzymes, and muscle symptoms are monitored and evaluated by a physician.

Red Yeast Rice Summary

TC	LDL-C	TG	HDL-C	Daily Dose	Safety	Interactions
Decrease	-21% to -32%	-13% to -44%	No effect	1200 – 3600 mg	Ensure Citrinin-free	Potential

References

Banach et al. 2018. The Role of Nutraceuticals in Statin Intolerant Patients: Position Paper from an International Lipid Expert Panel. J Am Coll Cardiol 2018; 72:96–118.

Cicero, A. F., A. Colletti, G. Bajraktari, O. Descamps, D. M. Djuric, M. Ezhov, Z. Fras, N. Katsiki, M. Langlois, G. Latkovskis, et al. 2017. Lipid lowering nutraceuticals in clinical practice: position paper from an International Lipid Expert Panel. Archives of Medical Science 13:965–1005.

Gordon RY, W. Obermeyer, T. Cooperman, and D. J. Becker. 2010. Marked variability of monacolin levels in commercial red yeast rice products. Arch Intern Med. 2010;170(19):1722–27.

Li Y., L. Jiang, Z. Jia, et al. 2014. A meta-analysis of red yeast rice: an effective and relatively safe alternative approach for dyslipidemia. PLoS One. 2014:9:e98611.

Rundek, T., A. Naini, R. Sacco, K. Coates, and S. DiMauro. Atorvastatin decreases the coenzyme Q10 level in the blood of patients at risk for cardiovascular disease and stroke. Arch. Neurol. 2004, 61, 889–892.

Shamim S, F. J. Al Badarin, J. J. DiNicolantonio, C. J. Lavie, and J. H. O'Keefe. 2013. Red yeast rice for dyslipidemia. *Missouri Medicine* 2013;110(4):349-54.

Thaipitakwong, T. and P. Aramwit. 2017. A review of the efficacy, safety, and clinical implications of naturally derived dietary supplements for dyslipidemia. American Journal of Cardiovascular Drugs. 2017 Feb;17(1):27-35.

CHAPTER 4

Bergamot

What is it?

Bergamot (*Citrus bergamia*) is a plant-based nutraceutical. Bergamot differs from other citrus fruits in its composition as it is rich in flavonoids that are related to its ability to lower cholesterol.

Effectiveness and Recommended Dose

Bergamot has been shown to be effective in reducing levels of LDL-C and TG. HDL-C levels were reported to be significantly increased.

Daily doses of 500 to 1000 mg/d of bergamot (bergamot derived polyphenolic fraction, BPF) have been shown in randomized clinical trials to reduce LDL-C levels by 15 – 40%. It was noted that the main limitation of evidence related to effectiveness is that most of the clinical literature has been provided by a single research lab and has not been confirmed elsewhere.

How does it work?

The flavonoids present in bergamot act as statins reducing the formation and transport of cholesterol. Increased fecal excretion may also be a mechanism of action. Bergamot may also inhibit the oxidation of LDL-C.

Safety Concerns and Upper Limits

Bergamot has a good safety profile and no side effects have been reported in clinical studies.

Interactions with medications

No information was identified concerning interactions of bergamot with medications. However, based on the similarity in mechanism of action to statins, caution should be used when taking bergamot at the same time as prescription statins.

Bergamot Summary

TC	LDL-C	TG	HDL-C	Daily Dose	Safety	Interactions
Decrease	-15% to -40%	Decrease	Increase	500 to 1000 mg	No side effects reported	Not available

References

Banach et al. 2018. The Role of Nutraceuticals in Statin Intolerant Patients: Position Paper from an International Lipid Expert Panel. J Am Coll Cardiol 2018; 72:96–118.

Cicero, A. F., A. Colletti, G. Bajraktari, O. Descamps, D. M. Djuric, M. Ezhov, Z. Fras, N. Katsiki, M. Langlois, G. Latkovskis, et al. 2017. Lipid lowering nutraceuticals in clinical practice: position paper from an International Lipid Expert Panel. *Archives of Medical Science* 13:965–1005.

Gliozzi, M., et al. 2013. Bergamot Polyphenolic Fraction Enhances Rosuvastatin-Induced Effect on LDL-Cholesterol, LOX-1 Expression and Protein Kinase B Phosphorylation in Patients with Hyperlipidemia. *International Journal of Cardiology*, 170, 140-145. http://dx.doi.org/10.1016/j.ijcard.2013.08.125

Gliozzi, M., *et al.* 2014. The Effect of Bergamot-Derived Polyphenolic Fraction on LDL Small Dense Particles and Non Alcoholic Fatty Liver Disease in Patients with Metabolic Syndrome. *Advances in Biological Chemistry*, 4,129-137. http://dx.doi.org/10.4236/abc.2014.42017

CHAPTER 5

Berberine

What is it?

Berberine is a plant-based nutraceutical found in many different plants including Chinese goldthread (*Coptis*), Goldenseal (*Hydrastis canadensis*), and Barberry (*Berberis*). Its chemical composition is a plant alkaloid related to its ability to lower cholesterol.

Effectiveness and Recommended Dose

Berberine has been shown to be effective in reducing levels of TC, LDL-C and TG. HDL-C levels were also reported to be increased.

Daily doses of 500 to 1500 mg/d of berberine have been shown in randomized clinical trials to reduce LDL-C levels by 15 – 20%.

How does it work?

Berberine acts on the LDL receptor in the liver. Secondary mechanisms of action may include a reduction in the intestinal absorption of cholesterol and increased fecal excretion of cholesterol.

Safety Concerns and Upper Limits

Side effects are mild to moderate gastrointestinal discomfort. No differences were observed in blood enzymes levels in comparison to control groups of the clinical trials.

Interactions with medications

No information was identified concerning interactions of berberine with medications.

Berberine Summary

TC	LDL-C	TG	HDL-C	Daily Dose	Safety	Interactions
Decrease	-15% to -20%	Decrease	Increase	500 to 1500 mg	Minimal side effects	Not available

References

Banach et al. 2018. The Role of Nutraceuticals in Statin Intolerant Patients: Position Paper from an International Lipid Expert Panel. J Am Coll Cardiol 2018; 72:96–118.

Cicero, A. F., A. Colletti, G. Bajraktari, O. Descamps, D. M. Djuric, M. Ezhov, Z. Fras, N. Katsiki, M. Langlois, G. Latkovskis, et al. 2017. Lipid lowering nutraceuticals in clinical practice: position paper from an International Lipid Expert Panel. Archives of Medical Science 13:965–1005.

CHAPTER 6

Fish Oil

What is it?

Fish oil is an animal-based nutraceutical derived from fish. It is enriched with eicosapentaenoic acid (EPA) and docosahexaenoic acid (DHA) which are omega-3 fatty acids.

Effectiveness and Recommended Dose

Fish oil is widely recommended and has been shown to be effective in reducing levels of TG by 18 to 25%. No effect on TC, LDL-C and HDL-C levels has been observed.

Daily doses of 1 to 4 g/d of fish oil have been shown in many randomized clinical trials to reduce TG levels. The EFSA determined in 2010 that intake of at least 2 g/d of DHA and EPA can maintain normal blood levels of TG. The AHA indicated that does of 2 to 4 g/d of EPA/DHA can reduce TG levels by 25-30%. It appears that fish oil exhibits dose-dependent effects with a higher reduction of TG reported for doses of 4 g/d or more. Doses lower than 2 to 4 g/d such as that found in margarine products (400 mg/d EPA/DHA) do not significantly reduce TG levels. Fish oil has also been associated with a significantly decreased rate of vascular death but did not have an impact on overall CVD endpoints or total mortality.

How does it work?

Fish oil inhibits the synthesis and turnover rate of TG. Additional benefits of fish oil include significant reductions in vascular stiffness and circulating inflammatory markers.

Safety Concerns and Upper Limits

Dose-dependent side effects have included body odor, bleeding, impaired immune function, increased lipid peroxidation, and impaired lipid and glucose metabolism. Most side effects are mild fishy aftertaste and gastrointestinal effects. People with allergies to seafood should avoid fish oil. The EFSA has determined that supplemental intakes of EPA and DHA combined at doses up to 5 g/d, supplemental intakes of EPA alone up to 1.8 g/d, and supplemental intakes of DHA alone up to 1 g/d do not raise safety concerns for adults. The FDA recommends an upper limit intake of 3 g/day of omega-3 fatty acids (EPA and DHA) as a safeguard against possible adverse effects. For those people using higher doses to lower TG should be under the care of a physician as bleeding and possible effects on immune function could occur. Pregnant or breastfeeding women should not take fish oil supplements due to the potential risk of mercury or other environmental contaminants.

Interactions with medications

Fish oil may interfere with Warfarin, anticoagulants, antihypertensives, and antiplatelets medications.

Fish Oil Summary

TC	LDL-C	TG	HDL-C	Daily Dose	Safety	Interactions
No effect	No effect	-18 to -30%	No effect	1 to 4 g	Minimal dose-dependent side effects	Potential

References

Banach et al. 2018. The Role of Nutraceuticals in Statin Intolerant Patients: Position Paper from an International Lipid Expert Panel. J Am Coll Cardiol 2018; 72:96–118.

Cicero, A. F., A. Colletti, G. Bajraktari, O. Descamps, D. M. Djuric, M. Ezhov, Z. Fras, N. Katsiki, M. Langlois, G. Latkovskis, et al. 2017. Lipid lowering nutraceuticals in clinical practice: position paper from an International Lipid Expert Panel. Archives of Medical Science 13:965–1005.

EFSA Panel on Dietetic Products, Nutrition and Allergies (NDA) 2012. Scientific Opinion related to the Tolerable Upper Intake Level of eicosapentaenoic acid (EPA), docosahexaenoic acid (DHA) and docosapentaenoic acid (DPA). EFSA Journal 2012;10(7):2815. [48 pp.] doi: 10.2903/j.efsa.2012.2815. Available online: www.efsa.europa.eu/efsajournal

National Institutes of Health, Office of Dietary Supplements. March 2, 2018. Omega-3 Fatty Acids Fact Sheet for Health Professionals. https://ods.od.nih.gov/factsheets/Omega3FattyAcids-HealthProfessional/

Thaipitakwong, T. and P. Aramwit. 2017. A review of the efficacy, safety, and clinical implications of naturally derived dietary supplements for dyslipidemia. American Journal of Cardiovascular Drugs. 2017 Feb;17(1):27-35.

CHAPTER 7

Krill Oil

What is it?

Krill oil is an animal-based nutraceutical derived from Antartic krill (*Euphausia superba*), a small crustacean. Like fish oil, it is enriched with EPA and DHA which are omega-3 fatty acids.

Effectiveness and Recommended Dose

Krill oil has been shown to be effective in reducing levels of TG by 10.2%. A small number of randomized clinical trials have reported a significant reduction of LDL-C (-15.52 mg/dl), TG (-14.03 mg/dl), and significant elevation of HDL-C (+6.65 mg/dl) levels.

At the same dose, krill oil appears to be more effective than fish oil. For example, a dose of 543 mg of DHA and EPA from krill oil was reported to be comparable to doses of 2.66 g of EPA and DHA present in fish oil.

How does it work?

Similar to fish oil, krill oil inhibits the synthesis and turnover rate of TG. The omega-3 fatty acids in krill oil appear to be better absorbed than that found in fish oil. This may be related to the high (40%) phosphatidylcholine content in krill oil which binds EPA and DHA resulting in an increase in therapeutic efficacy.

Safety Concerns and Upper Limits

No significant adverse effects have been reported in clinical trials. A small increase in the enzyme gamma-glutamyl transferase, an indicator of liver function, was reported. The EFSA has determined that supplemental intakes of EPA and DHA combined at doses up to 5 g/d, supplemental intakes of EPA alone up to 1.8 g/d, and supplemental intakes of DHA alone up to 1 g/d do not raise safety concerns for adults. The FDA recommends an upper limit intake of 3 g/day of omega-3 fatty acids (EPA and DHA) as a safeguard against possible adverse effects. For those people using higher doses to lower TG should be under the care of a physician as bleeding and possible effects on immune function could occur. Pregnant or breastfeeding women should not take krill oil supplements due to the potential risk of mercury or other environmental contaminants.

Interactions with medications

Similar to fish oil, krill oil may interfere with Warfarin, anticoagulants, antihypertensives, and antiplatelets medications.

Krill Oil Summary

TC	LDL-C	TG	HDL-C	Daily Dose	Safety	Interactions
No effect	Decrease	-10.2%	Increase	500 mg to 4000 mg	Minimal dose-dependent side effects	Potential

References

Banach et al. 2018. The Role of Nutraceuticals in Statin Intolerant Patients: Position Paper from an International Lipid Expert Panel. J Am Coll Cardiol 2018; 72:96–118.

Cicero, A. F., A. Colletti, G. Bajraktari, O. Descamps, D. M. Djuric, M. Ezhov, Z. Fras, N. Katsiki, M. Langlois, G. Latkovskis, et al. 2017. Lipid lowering nutraceuticals in clinical practice: position paper from an International Lipid Expert Panel. Archives of Medical Science 13:965–1005.

EFSA Panel on Dietetic Products, Nutrition and Allergies (NDA) 2012. Scientific Opinion related to the Tolerable Upper Intake Level of eicosapentaenoic acid (EPA), docosahexaenoic acid (DHA) and docosapentaenoic acid (DPA). EFSA Journal 2012;10(7):2815. [48 pp.] doi: 10.2903/j.efsa.2012.2815. Available online: www.efsa.europa.eu/efsajournal

National Institutes of Health, Office of Dietary Supplements. March 2, 2018. Omega-3 Fatty Acids Fact Sheet for Health Professionals. https://ods.od.nih.gov/factsheets/Omega3FattyAcids-HealthProfessional/

Thaipitakwong, T. and P. Aramwit. 2017. A review of the efficacy, safety, and clinical implications of naturally derived dietary supplements for dyslipidemia. American Journal of Cardiovascular Drugs. 2017 Feb;17(1):27-35.

Ursoniu, S, A. Sahebkar, M.C. Serban, et al. (2017) Lipid-modifying effects of krill oil in humans: systematic review and meta-analysis of randomized controlled trials. Nutr Rev 75, 361–373.

CHAPTER 8

Phytosterols

What is it?

Phytosterols are plant-derived sterols and stanols that have been shown to be effective in the reduction of LDL-C levels. Plant sterols are present in many plant sources such as vegetable oils, nuts, seeds, legumes and fat spreads. The structure of plant sterols is similar to cholesterol. Because the average intake of plant sterols and stanols in most people's diet is low, supplementation may offer an alternative to lower cholesterol.

Effectiveness and Recommended Dose

Phytosterols have been shown to be effective in reducing levels of LDL-C.

A daily dose of 400 – 3000 mg/day of phytosterols has been shown in randomized clinical trials to reduce LDL-C levels by 8 - 12%. Additionally, the cholesterol lowering effect of phytosterols is dose-dependent with a plateau reached at approximately 3000 mg/day which achieved a reduction of LDL-C of 12%.

How does it work?

Phytosterols are believed to work by decreasing cholesterol absorption and enhancing the fecal excretion of bile acid and cholesterol.

Safety Concerns and Upper Limits

Phytosterols have a high safety profile at least in middle term studies. Some common side effects include gastrointestinal symptoms and decreased absorption of fat-soluble vitamins. A rare but serious condition has been reported in which phytosterols accumulate in the blood and tissues.

Interactions with medications

Phytosterols may increase the effects of ezetimibe a drug that lowers plasma cholesterol levels and share a similar mechanism of action.

Phytosterols Summary

TC	LDL-C	TG	HDL-C	Daily Dose	Safety	Interactions
-10% to -14%	-8% to -12%	No effect	No effect	400 to 3000 mg	Minimal side effects	Potential

References

Banach et al. 2018. The Role of Nutraceuticals in Statin Intolerant Patients: Position Paper from an International Lipid Expert Panel. J Am Coll Cardiol 2018; 72:96–118.

Cicero, A. F., A. Colletti, G. Bajraktari, O. Descamps, D. M. Djuric, M. Ezhov, Z. Fras, N. Katsiki, M. Langlois, G. Latkovskis, et al. 2017. Lipid lowering nutraceuticals in clinical practice: position paper from an International Lipid Expert Panel. Archives of Medical Science 13:965–1005.

Thaipitakwong, T. and P. Aramwit. 2017. A review of the efficacy, safety, and clinical implications of naturally derived dietary supplements for dyslipidemia. American Journal of Cardiovascular Drugs. 2017 Feb;17(1):27-35.

CHAPTER 9

Soluble Fiber

What is it?

Dietary fiber is found in a variety of plant-derived sources that do not undergo significant digestion in the gastrointestinal tract. Oats, psyllium, beans, and nuts are sources of soluble fiber that have been shown to lower cholesterol.

Effectiveness and Recommended Dose

Soluble fiber has been shown to be effective in reducing levels of total cholesterol TC and LDL-C. No effect on TG and HDL-C levels has been observed.

The reduction of cholesterol due to soluble fiber is variable and dependent on the type of fiber, doses, and study details. In general, TC reduction has been reported from 0 – 18% of oat-based fibers, 3-17% for psyllium, 5-16% for pectin, and 4-17% for guar gum.

Specific data has been reported for β-glucan, psyllium, and glucomannan. A daily dose of 3 g/day of β-glucan has been shown in randomized clinical trials to reduce LDL-C. A daily dose of 10 g/day of psyllium has been shown in randomized clinical trials to reduce LDL-C by 7%. A daily dose of 5 -15 g/day of glucomannan has been shown in randomized clinical trials to reduce LDL-C by 5 -15%.

How does it work?

Soluble fiber is believed to work by decreasing cholesterol absorption and enhancing the fecal excretion of bile acid and cholesterol.

Safety Concerns and Upper Limits

In general, soluble fiber has a good safety profile. A viscous gel forms after ingestion that delays intestinal mobility causing a decrease in cholesterol absorption and overall food consumption. This may lead to nausea, vomiting, and bloating which have been reported in clinical trials. Intestinal obstruction is also a possible long-term complication.

There are not enough data available for β-glucan to evaluate safety. A good safety profile has been reported for psyllium in clinical trials at doses up to 20 g/day. Some minor gastrointestinal side effects were reported. In general, glucomannan consumption does not cause serious side effects other than minor gastrointestinal effects.

Interactions with medications

Soluble fiber, and particularly glucomannan, may interfere with the absorption of certain fat-soluble drugs and nutraceuticals such as vitamin E, calcium and other minerals. To counteract this potential effect, it is recommended that the medication should be taken 1 hour before or at least 4 hours after taking glucomannan.

Soluble Fiber Summary

TC	LDL-C	TG	HDL-C	Daily Dose	Safety	Interactions
Decrease 0 to -18%	-5 to -15%	No effect	No effect	3 g β-glucan 10 g psyllium 5 -15 g glucomannan	Minimal side effects	Potential

References

Banach et al. 2018. The Role of Nutraceuticals in Statin Intolerant Patients: Position Paper from an International Lipid Expert Panel. J Am Coll Cardiol 2018; 72:96–118.

Cicero, A. F., A. Colletti, G. Bajraktari, O. Descamps, D. M. Djuric, M. Ezhov, Z. Fras, N. Katsiki, M. Langlois, G. Latkovskis, et al. 2017. Lipid lowering nutraceuticals in clinical practice: position paper from an International Lipid Expert Panel. Archives of Medical Science 13:965–1005.

Thaipitakwong, T. and P. Aramwit. 2017. A review of the efficacy, safety, and clinical implications of naturally derived dietary supplements for dyslipidemia. American Journal of Cardiovascular Drugs. 2017 Feb;17(1):27-35.

CHAPTER 10

Artichoke

What is it?

Artichoke (*Cynara cardunculus*) is a plant-based nutraceutical with antioxidant action. It has been demonstrated to lower cholesterol.

Effectiveness and Recommended Dose

Artichoke has been shown to be effective in reducing levels of TC, LDL-C, and TG. No effect on HDL-C levels has been observed.

Daily doses of 1 to 3 g of spirulina have been shown in randomized clinical trials to reduce LDL-C levels by 5 - 15%.

How does it work?

Artichoke is believed to work by interacting with the key enzyme involved in the natural synthesis of cholesterol causing a reduction of your body's natural production of cholesterol.

Safety Concerns and Upper Limits

No serious side effects have been reported in clinical trials indicating the tolerability and safety of artichoke in the short to medium term. In some cases, minor and short term gastrointestinal effects have been observed.

Interactions with medications

No information was identified concerning interactions of artichoke with medications.

Artichoke Summary

TC	LDL-C	TG	HDL-C	Daily Dose	Safety	Interactions
Decrease	-5 to -15%	Decrease	No effect	1 to 3 g	Minimal side effects	Not available

References

Banach et al. 2018. The Role of Nutraceuticals in Statin Intolerant Patients: Position Paper from an International Lipid Expert Panel. J Am Coll Cardiol 2018; 72:96–118.

Cicero, A. F., A. Colletti, G. Bajraktari, O. Descamps, D. M. Djuric, M. Ezhov, Z. Fras, N. Katsiki, M. Langlois, G. Latkovskis, et al. 2017. Lipid lowering nutraceuticals in clinical practice: position paper from an International Lipid Expert Panel. Archives of Medical Science 13:965–1005.

CHAPTER 11

Garlic

What is it?

Garlic (*Allium sativum*) is a plant-based nutraceutical that contains organosulfur compounds that are responsible for its medicinal properties. The primary component of garlic is called Allicin and is believed to be responsible for its lipid-lowering mechanism of action.

Effectiveness and Recommended Dose

Garlic has been shown to be effective in reducing levels of total cholesterol TC and LDL-C. No effect on TG levels but an increase in HDL-C levels has also been observed in clinical trials.

A daily dose of 6 g/day of garlic has been shown in randomized clinical trials to reduce LDL-C levels by 5 to 10%. The percentage of allicin available will affect the required dose for lowering cholesterol. Additional benefits of garlic are its lowering effect on blood pressure and antiplatelet effect.

How does it work?

Garlic is believed to work by inhibiting the key enzyme involved in the natural synthesis of cholesterol causing a reduction of your body's natural production of cholesterol. It may also block the absorption of dietary cholesterol and fatty acids and increase the excretion of bile acids in the liver.

Safety Concerns and Upper Limits

No serious adverse effects have been reported in clinical trials. However, many people experience unpleasant odor and aftertaste, and mild gastrointestinal symptoms such as nausea and bloating. The high doses required for garlic to be effective may limit the use of garlic to lower cholesterol due to its aftertaste.

Interactions with medications

Garlic may interfere with Warfarin, protease inhibitors (e.g., saquinavir), anticoagulants, antihypertensives, and antiplatelets medications.

Garlic Summary

TC	LDL-C	TG	HDL-C	Daily Dose	Safety	Interactions
Decrease	-5% to -10%	No effect	Increase	6 g	Minimal side effects	Potential

References

Banach et al. 2018. The Role of Nutraceuticals in Statin Intolerant Patients: Position Paper from an International Lipid Expert Panel. J Am Coll Cardiol 2018; 72:96–118.

Cicero, A. F., A. Colletti, G. Bajraktari, O. Descamps, D. M. Djuric, M. Ezhov, Z. Fras, N. Katsiki, M. Langlois, G. Latkovskis, et al. 2017. Lipid lowering nutraceuticals in clinical practice: position paper from an International Lipid Expert Panel. Archives of Medical Science 13:965–1005.

Thaipitakwong, T. and P. Aramwit. 2017. A review of the efficacy, safety, and clinical implications of naturally derived dietary supplements for dyslipidemia. American Journal of Cardiovascular Drugs. 2017 Feb;17(1):27-35.

CHAPTER 12

Rice Bran Oil

What is it?

Rice bran oil is a plant-based nutraceutical. Gamma-oryzanol (γ-oryzanol) is the primary bioactive component that is related to its ability to lower cholesterol. Different percentages of γ-oryzanol are in rice bran oil with a reported range of 27.7 to 61.6 mg/100g).

Effectiveness and Recommended Dose

γ-oryzanol has been shown to be effective in reducing levels of TC and LDL-C. HDL-C levels were also reported to be increased, but only in men.

Daily doses of 300 mg/d of γ-oryzanol have been shown in randomized clinical trials to reduce LDL-C levels by 5 – 10%.

How does it work?

γ-oryzanol works by inhibiting the key enzyme involved in the natural synthesis of cholesterol and reducing intestinal absorption. This results in a reduction of your body's natural production of cholesterol. This is a similar mechanism to statin prescription drugs.

Safety Concerns and Upper Limits

No side effects have been reported with rice bran oil consumption.

Interactions with medications

No information was identified concerning interactions of rice bran oil with medications. However, based on the similarity in mechanism of action to statins, caution should be used when taking rice bran oil at the same time as prescription statins.

Rice Bran Oil Summary

TC	LDL-C	TG	HDL-C	Daily Dose	Safety	Interactions
Decrease	-5% to -10%	No effect	Increase (men only)	300 mg	No side effects reported	Not available

References

Banach et al. 2018. The Role of Nutraceuticals in Statin Intolerant Patients: Position Paper from an International Lipid Expert Panel. J Am Coll Cardiol 2018; 72:96–118.

Cicero, A. F., A. Colletti, G. Bajraktari, O. Descamps, D. M. Djuric, M. Ezhov, Z. Fras, N. Katsiki, M. Langlois, G. Latkovskis, et al. 2017. Lipid lowering nutraceuticals in clinical practice: position paper from an International Lipid Expert Panel. Archives of Medical Science 13:965–1005.

CHAPTER 13

Soy Protein

What is it?

Soy (*Glycine max*) is a plant-based nutraceutical which has bioactive compounds that may be responsible for its lipid lowering effect.

Effectiveness and Recommended Dose

Soy protein has been shown to be effective in reducing levels of total cholesterol TC, LDL-C, and TG. An increase in HDL-C levels has also been observed in clinical trials.

A daily dose of 25 – 100 g/day of soy protein has been shown in randomized clinical trials to reduce LDL-C levels by 3 to 10%. Additional benefits of soy protein may include the attenuation of inflammatory processes and atherosclerotic plaque formation, and improvements in vascular function.

How does it work?

Soy protein is believed to work by decreasing cholesterol absorption and enhancing the fecal excretion of bile acid and cholesterol.

Safety Concerns and Upper Limits

Skin allergic reactions, constipation, bloating, and nausea have been reported in clinical trials. Chronic use of high quantities of soy products could affect thyroid function and fertility as well as reduce the absorption of minerals such as calcium, magnesium, copper, iron, and zinc. The long-term use of soy isoflavone supplements, which have estrogenic activity, could increase the risk of thickening of the lining of the uterus that may lead to cancer. It appears that it is safe for women who have breast cancer or who are at risk for breast cancer to eat soy foods, but it is uncertain whether soy isoflavone supplements are safe for these women. The high dose required to reduce cholesterol may limit the use of soy protein.

Interactions with medications

No information was identified concerning interactions of soy protein with medications.

Soy Protein Summary

TC	LDL-C	TG	HDL-C	Daily Dose	Safety	Interactions
Decrease	-3% to -10%	Decrease	Increase	25 to 100g	Moderate side effects; Soy isoflavone caution	No information

References

Banach et al. 2018. The Role of Nutraceuticals in Statin Intolerant Patients: Position Paper from an International Lipid Expert Panel. J Am Coll Cardiol 2018; 72:96–118.

Cicero, A. F., A. Colletti, G. Bajraktari, O. Descamps, D. M. Djuric, M. Ezhov, Z. Fras, N. Katsiki, M. Langlois, G. Latkovskis, et al. 2017. Lipid lowering nutraceuticals in clinical practice: position paper from an International Lipid Expert Panel. Archives of Medical Science 13:965–1005.

National Institutes of Health (NIH), National Center for Complementary and Integrative Health. 2016. Soy. https://nccih.nih.gov/health/soy/ataglance.htm

Thaipitakwong, T. and P. Aramwit. 2017. A review of the efficacy, safety, and clinical implications of naturally derived dietary supplements for dyslipidemia. American Journal of Cardiovascular Drugs. 2017 Feb;17(1):27-35.

CHAPTER 14

Green Tea

What is it?

Green tea (*Camellia sinensis*) is a plant-based nutraceutical which is rich in antioxidants such as polyphenols that may be responsible for its lipid lowering effect.

Effectiveness and Recommended Dose

Green tea and its extracts have been shown to be effective in reducing levels of total cholesterol TC and LDL-C. No effect on TG and HDL-C levels has been observed.

A daily dose of 250 – 1200 mg/day of green tea extract has been shown in randomized clinical trials to reduce LDL-C levels by 5%. Additional benefits of green may include improvements in vascular function.

How does it work?

Green tea is believed to work by decreasing cholesterol absorption and enhancing the fecal excretion of bile acid and cholesterol.

Safety Concerns and Upper Limits

In general, the consumption of green tea is well tolerated. Some effects have been noted and include rash, short-term elevation of blood pressure, and mild gastrointestinal disorders. Adverse effects related to the effects of caffeine are also possible. High doses of green tea could cause a deficiency of iron and folate because of a reduction of intestinal absorption. Due to liver problems in a small number of people who took concentrated green tea extracts, it has been recommended that concentrated green tea extracts be taken with food and that use be discontinued if symptoms of a liver disorder persist. A reduction in the blood levels of the drug nadolol, a beta-blocker used for high blood pressure and heart problems has also been reported.

Interactions with medications

Green tea may interfere with Warfarin, anticoagulants and antiplatelets medications.

Green Tea Summary

TC	LDL-C	TG	HDL-C	Daily Dose	Safety	Interactions
Decrease	-5%	No effect	No effect	250 to 1200 mg	Minimal side effects	Potential

References

Banach et al. 2018. The Role of Nutraceuticals in Statin Intolerant Patients: Position Paper from an International Lipid Expert Panel. J Am Coll Cardiol 2018; 72:96–118.

Cicero, A. F., A. Colletti, G. Bajraktari, O. Descamps, D. M. Djuric, M. Ezhov, Z. Fras, N. Katsiki, M. Langlois, G. Latkovskis, et al. 2017. Lipid lowering nutraceuticals in clinical practice: position paper from an International Lipid Expert Panel. Archives of Medical Science 13:965–1005.

National Institutes of Health (NIH), National Center for Complementary and Integrative Health. 2016. Green Tea. https://nccih.nih.gov/health/greentea

Thaipitakwong, T. and P. Aramwit. 2017. A review of the efficacy, safety, and clinical implications of naturally derived dietary supplements for dyslipidemia. American Journal of Cardiovascular Drugs. 2017 Feb;17(1):27-35.

CHAPTER 15

Chitosan

What is it?

Chitosan is derived from chitin which is a component of the shells of crustaceans. Chitosan has been shown to lower cholesterol.

Effectiveness and Recommended Dose

Chitosan has been shown to be effective in reducing levels of TC and LDL-C.

A daily dose of 1 - 6 g/day of chitosan has been shown in randomized clinical trials to reduce LDL-C levels by 5%. However, some studies were inconsistent and only showed a significant reduction in TC levels.

How does it work?

Chitosan is believed to work by decreasing the intestinal absorption of cholesterol.

Safety Concerns and Upper Limits

Although some changes in safety parameters have been observed, none were clinically meaningful. Short-term sides effects such as abdominal pain, diarrhea, vomiting, and constipation have been reported in rare cases at doses of 1 – 6 g/day.

Interactions with medications

Chitosan may interfere with Warfarin, anticoagulants and antiplatelets medications.

Chitosan Summary

TC	LDL-C	TG	HDL-C	Daily Dose	Safety	Interactions
Decrease	-5%	No effect	No effect	1 to 6 g	Minimal side effects	Potential

References

Cicero, A. F., A. Colletti, G. Bajraktari, O. Descamps, D. M. Djuric, M. Ezhov, Z. Fras, N. Katsiki, M. Langlois, G. Latkovskis, et al. 2017. Lipid lowering nutraceuticals in clinical practice: position paper from an International Lipid Expert Panel. Archives of Medical Science 13:965–1005.

Thaipitakwong, T. and P. Aramwit. 2017. A review of the efficacy, safety, and clinical implications of naturally derived dietary supplements for dyslipidemia. American Journal of Cardiovascular Drugs. 2017 Feb;17(1):27-35.

CHAPTER 16

Spirulina

What is it?

Spirulina (*Arthrospira platensis*) is a plant-based nutraceutical which is derived from filamentous microalga. Spirulina has high amounts of antioxidants and has been demonstrated to lower cholesterol.

Effectiveness and Recommended Dose

Spirulina has been shown to be effective in reducing levels of TC, LDL-C, and TG. HDL-C levels were also reported to be increased.

Daily doses of 1 to 10 g of spirulina have been shown in randomized clinical trials to reduce LDL-C levels by 5%.

How does it work?

The mechanism of action of spirulina is unclear but may be related to the high amounts of antioxidants.

Safety Concerns and Upper Limits

Spirulina appears to be safe and well tolerated.

Interactions with medications

No information was identified concerning interactions of spirulina with medications.

Spirulina Summary

TC	LDL-C	TG	HDL-C	Daily Dose	Safety	Interactions
Decrease	-5%	Decrease	Increase	1 to 10 g	No side effects reported	Not available

References

Banach et al. 2018. The Role of Nutraceuticals in Statin Intolerant Patients: Position Paper from an International Lipid Expert Panel. J Am Coll Cardiol 2018; 72:96–118.

Cicero, A. F., A. Colletti, G. Bajraktari, O. Descamps, D. M. Djuric, M. Ezhov, Z. Fras, N. Katsiki, M. Langlois, G. Latkovskis, et al. 2017. Lipid lowering nutraceuticals in clinical practice: position paper from an International Lipid Expert Panel. Archives of Medical Science 13:965–1005.

CHAPTER 17

Probiotics

What is it?

Probiotics are microorganisms that have health benefits. Specific bacteria such as *Bifidobacterium* and *Lactobacillus* are common in probiotics. Probiotics have been shown to lower cholesterol.

Effectiveness and Recommended Dose

Probiotics have been shown to be effective in reducing levels of total cholesterol TC and LDL-C. No effect on TG and HDL-C levels has been observed.

The daily dose of probiotics is bacteria-strain dependent but has been shown in randomized clinical trials to reduce LDL-C levels by 5%. Available studies suggest that *Lactobacillus* strains are most effective at cholesterol reduction. So far, clinical results are not sufficient to support a recommendation as a non-drug alternative for cholesterol control.

How does it work?

Probiotics are believed to work by decreasing the intestinal absorption of cholesterol and enhancing the fecal excretion of bile acid and cholesterol. Lactobacillus contain some enzymes that transform cholesterol into a form that can be excreted in the feces. Some other probiotics have been shown to increase the excretion of bile acids.

Safety Concerns and Upper Limits

Probiotics have been safe and well tolerated in short-term clinical trials.

Interactions with medications

No information was identified concerning interactions of probiotics with medications.

Probiotics Summary

TC	LDL-C	TG	HDL-C	Daily Dose	Safety	Interactions
Decrease	-5%	No effect	No effect	Bacteria-strain dependent	No effects reported	Not available

References

Banach et al. 2018. The Role of Nutraceuticals in Statin Intolerant Patients: Position Paper from an International Lipid Expert Panel. J Am Coll Cardiol 2018; 72:96–118.

Cicero, A. F., A. Colletti, G. Bajraktari, O. Descamps, D. M. Djuric, M. Ezhov, Z. Fras, N. Katsiki, M. Langlois, G. Latkovskis, et al. 2017. Lipid lowering nutraceuticals in clinical practice: position paper from an International Lipid Expert Panel. Archives of Medical Science 13:965–1005.

Thaipitakwong, T. and P. Aramwit. 2017. A review of the efficacy, safety, and clinical implications of naturally derived dietary supplements for dyslipidemia. American Journal of Cardiovascular Drugs. 2017 Feb;17(1):27-35.

CHAPTER 18

Flaxseed

What is it?

Flaxseed (*Linum usitatissimum*) is a plant-based nutraceutical usually in the form of ground seed or oil. Alpha-linolenic acid (ALA), a plant-based omega-3 fatty acid, is a primary component of flaxseed. Flaxseed has been shown to lower cholesterol.

Effectiveness and Recommended Dose

Flaxseed has been shown to be effective in reducing levels of total cholesterol TC and LDL-C. No effect on TG and HDL-C levels has been observed.

Daily doses of 20.0 to 50.0 g/d (median dose: 38.0 g) of flaxseed have been shown in randomized clinical trials to reduce LDL-C levels. It was noted that the beneficial effects of flaxseed and its derivatives were only observed among those with relatively high initial cholesterol concentrations.

How does it work?

Flaxseed is believed to work by inhibiting cholesterol and fatty acid production in the liver through the suppression of gene expression. Other potential mechanisms of action include blocking intestinal cholesterol absorption due to high fiber content.

Safety Concerns and Upper Limits

Minimal side effects have been observed in clinical trials. Flaxseed could cause gastrointestinal discomfort and potentially intestinal blockage.

Interactions with medications

Flaxseed may interfere with the absorption of certain fat-soluble drugs and nutraceuticals such as vitamin E, calcium and other minerals. It may also interfere with Warfarin, anticoagulants, antihypertensives, and antiplatelets medications.

Flaxseed Summary

TC	LDL-C	TG	HDL-C	Daily Dose	Safety	Interactions
Decrease	Decrease	No effect	No effect	20.0 to 50.0 g (median dose: 38.0 g)	Minimal side effects	Potential

References

Pan, A, D. Yu, W. Demark-Wahnefried, et al. (2009) Meta-analysis of the effects of flaxseed interventions on blood lipids. Am J Clin Nutr 90, 288–297.

Thaipitakwong, T. and P. Aramwit. 2017. A review of the efficacy, safety, and clinical implications of naturally derived dietary supplements for dyslipidemia. American Journal of Cardiovascular Drugs. 2017 Feb;17(1):27-35.

CHAPTER 19

Other Dietary Supplements with Limited Effectiveness

Several dietary supplements have been cited as having lipid-lowering effects. Below is a list of dietary supplements with limited effectiveness. Until additional clinical studies have been performed to clarify lipid-lowering potential and safety considerations, these supplements are not recommended.

Dietary Supplement	Comments
Anthocyanins	One Study of Diabetic Patients
Astaxanthin	Not Supported by Clinical Evidence
L-Carnitine	Non-significant Results
Conjugated Linoleic Acid	Limited Studies; Potential Impairment of Endothelial Function
Curcumin	Inconsistent Efficacy; Low Oral Bioavailability
Guggulipids	Inconsistent Efficacy; Elevation of LDL-C
Hibiscus sabdarrifa (sour tea)	Effects not Substantiated
Lecithin	Limited Clinical Data with Small Sample Size
Pantetheine	Limited Efficacy
Policosanols	Inconsistent Efficacy; Non-significant Results
Resveratrol	Effects not Substantiated

Sesame (Sesamum indicum)	Inconsistent Efficacy
Silymarin	Data not available; Low Bioavailability
Vitamin E	Minimal Effects

References

Cicero, A. F., A. Colletti, G. Bajraktari, O. Descamps, D. M. Djuric, M. Ezhov, Z. Fras, N. Katsiki, M. Langlois, G. Latkovskis, et al. 2017. Lipid lowering nutraceuticals in clinical practice: position paper from an International Lipid Expert Panel. Archives of Medical Science 13:965–1005.

A. M. Mourad, E. de Carvalho Pincinato, P. G. Mazzola, M. Sabha, and P. Moriel. 2010. Influence of soy lecithin administration on hypercholesterolemia, Cholesterol, 2010, 824813.

Thaipitakwong, T. and P. Aramwit. 2017. A review of the efficacy, safety, and clinical implications of naturally derived dietary supplements for dyslipidemia. American Journal of Cardiovascular Drugs. 2017 Feb;17(1):27-35.

CHAPTER 20

Summary and Recommended Approach

The effectiveness of dietary supplements for cholesterol control may be modest or have no effect. Therefore, even with the best supplement to lower cholesterol, it should be combined with a healthy diet, regular physical activity, and positive lifestyle changes.

As summarized in the previous chapters, dietary supplements can have significant safety concerns. Don't assume that dietary supplements are safe because they are "natural." If a dietary supplement can lower your blood cholesterol there can also be other effects in your body.

Many of the dietary supplements included in this book might have non–lipid-lowering actions, including improvement of endothelial dysfunction and arterial stiffness, as well as anti-inflammatory and antioxidative properties. These include RYR, Green Tea, Soy Protein, Fish Oil, and Krill Oil.

My personal experience has shown that approximately 2400 mg of RYR in divided doses, 1000 mg EPA +DHA from fish oil, and 350 mg krill oil (50 mg EPA +24 mg DHA) has been most effective at improving my lipid profile. Lecithin was not effective at improving my LDL-C levels but did have a lowering effect on TG. I have not evaluated other dietary supplements and, therefore, cannot provide perspective on their potential effectiveness.

A recommended plan for utilizing dietary supplements for lowering cholesterol is summarized below.

- Consult with your personal physician on the dietary supplements that you consider taking.

- Conduct your own research for the selection of a dietary supplement that includes a review of clinical studies that demonstrate effectiveness and dose to use as well as safety considerations.

- Before taking a dietary supplement, have your blood lipid levels tested to establish a baseline upon which to gauge the effectiveness of dietary supplements and for safety considerations.

- Evaluate any potential interactions with the prescription drugs or other dietary supplements that you are taking.

- Only take one dietary supplement at a time to determine its effectiveness. If desired cholesterol levels are not obtained, additional supplements should be added one at a time as well to determine the combined effect.

- If you have any obvious side effects from taking a dietary supplement, immediately discontinue use.

- Do not take more than the upper intake limit (if established). The lowest effective dose may help minimize side effects.

- Retest your blood lipid levels after 3 months of use of the dietary supplement. Evaluate changes in your blood lipids as well as blood enzyme levels that could be indicative of liver or kidney function. Consider other factors that could affect your lipid profile such as weight change and other lifestyle factors that could affect cholesterol levels. Annual blood lipid level testing will ensure that effectiveness is consistent and allow for screening of potential adverse effects.

- If desired cholesterol levels are not obtained, consider trying another dietary supplement that has a different mechanism of action. Consider the brand and formulation of the dietary supplement that was used as wide variability can exist.

- Dietary supplements should only be one part of your personal health plan. A healthy diet, regular exercise, maintenance of a healthy body weight, healthy lifestyle, and medications prescribed by your doctor should all be considered as parts of your plan.

www.ingramcontent.com/pod-product-compliance
Lightning Source LLC
Chambersburg PA
CBHW061737250726
48657CB00002B/965